Kickboxing

Fitness

A Guide for

Fitness

Professionals

from the

American

Council

on Exercise

Second Edition

By Tony Ordas, M.A.,

and Tim Rochford

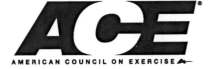

AMERICAN COUNCIL ON EXERCISE

First edition

Copyright © 2004 American Council on Exercise (ACE)

Printed in the United States of America.

ABCDE

ISBN: 1-58518-916-2

Library of Congress Control Number: 2004113368

Distributed by:

American Council on Exercise

P.O. Box 910449

San Diego, CA 92191-0449

(858) 279-8227

(858) 279-8064 (FAX)

www.ACEfitness.org

Managing Editor: Daniel J. Green
Technical Editor: Cedric X. Bryant, Ph.D.
Design & Production: Karen McGuire
Director of Publications: Christine J. Ekeroth
Assistant Editor: Jennifer Schiffer
Index: Bonny McLaughlin
Models: Joe Jimenez, Frank Luna, Tony Ordas, & Dawn Rosemier
Photography: Dennis Dal Covey

Acknowledgments:

Thanks to the entire American Council on Exercise staff for their support and guidance through the process of creating this manual.

NOTICE

The fitness industry is ever-changing. As new research and clinical experience broaden our knowledge, changes in programming and standards are required. The authors and the publisher of this work have checked with sources believed to be reliable in their efforts to provide information that is complete and generally in accord with the standards accepted at the time of publication. However, in view of the possibility of human error or changes in industry standards, neither the authors nor the publisher nor any other party who has been involved in the preparation or publication of this work warrants that the information contained herein is in every respect accurate or complete, and they are not responsible for any errors or omissions or the results obtained from the use of such information. Readers are encouraged to confirm the information contained herein with other sources.

Published by:

Healthy Learning Books & Videos

P.O. Box 1828

Monterey, CA 93942

(888) 229-5745

(831) 372-6075 (Fax)

www.healthylearning.com

P04-038

Linda Dunn, M.A., is an ACE-certified Group Fitness Instructor and Personal Trainer and an ACSM-certified Exercise Leader. She is the recreation director for the First United Methodist Church in Tuscaloosa, Ala., and an aerobics and yoga instructor at several local facilities. Dunn is also a personal trainer specializing in working with children and older adults at the North River Yacht Club.

Jackie Hawkins Lynds, B.S., is ACE-certified and CHEK II-certified as a Personal Trainer. She is a Certified BoxAerobic Instructor, a black belt in Kenpo Karate, and a personal trainer with Frog's Club One in La Jolla, Calif.

Sifu Richard Scott has 36 years of experience in the martial arts. He is a 5th Degree Black Belt in Kenpo Karate and was the owner and head instructor at Arena Martial Arts in San Diego, Calif. He is currently teaching and training with Cepeda-Abueg Martial Arts and is a certified USA Boxing Coach with experience in boxing, kickboxing, Kali, Arnis de Mano, Jiu-Jitsu, Aikido, and Tae Kwon Do. Scott has trained three California State Kickboxing Champions, two California State Women's Boxing Champions, and one National Golden Glove Champion in the women's division.

Joseph Signorile, Ph.D., is an associate professor of exercise physiology at the University of Miami and researcher at the Miami Veteran's Affairs Medical Center, and the exercise science and sports medicine director for the International Sports Conditioning Association and Promise Enterprises. He is a member of the American College of Sports Medicine, the National Strength and Conditioning Association, and the American Physiological Society. Dr. Signorile is extensively published in the areas of training theory, aging and training, and sports-specific conditioning.

Kathy Yeh, M.A., is an exercise physiologist and a 3rd Dan in Tae Kwon Do. She has been training in Tae Kwon Do for 20 years and also has experience in Tang Soo Do, Capoeira, boxing, and short sticks. She was bronze medalist both at the Tae Kwon Do Nationals and the Olympic Festival in 1991. Yeh is an ACE-certified Personal Trainer and ACSM-certified health and fitness instructor, and has served on the ACE Personal Trainer Exam Committee.

The authors would also like to thank Sifu Steve Eckberg, Sifu/Kru Frank Navarro, Tricia Baglio Alker, and Randy Ballard for their contributions to this book.

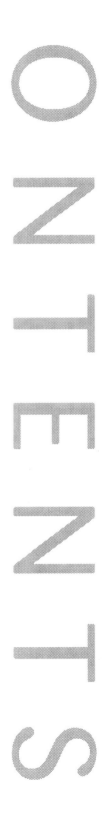

The American Council on Exercise (ACE) is pleased to introduce *Kickboxing Fitness,* a guide for fitness professionals. Kickboxing has long been a popular mode of group exercise, and it continues to be a favorite among personal trainers as well. The purpose of this book is to provide guidelines and criteria so that this exercise modality can be practiced both safely and effectively, and to educate and give guidance to fitness professionals that wish to teach kickboxing. As with all areas of fitness, education is a continual process. ACE recognizes this is a broad subject requiring serious study and we encourage you to use the References and Suggested Reading to further your knowledge.

INTRODUCTION

Introduction to Kickboxing Fitness

Kickboxing, which is rooted in Western boxing and Muay Thai (Thai kickboxing), can be traced as far back as 5000 years ago to boxing in the Middle East. Its popularity spread throughout the Mediterranean to Ancient Greece and the Roman Empire, but the sport was eventually banned because of its brutality. There were no breaks in the action and fights were bloody. Competitors used open-hand strikes and blocks as well as leg strikes using the knees, shins, and feet. These matches were stopped only when an opponent was either knocked out or killed.

CHAPTER ONE

The sport disappeared from the public eye until 1719, when James Figg, a fighter and teacher, revived the sport by featuring men and women boxing as a spectator event in London. Opponents fought bare-knuckled and were allowed to kick, catch-hold-hit, scratch, wrestle, maul, and throw their opponents. To help promote gambling at these matches, Jack Broughton, known as the father of modern boxing, and Captain John Godfrey wrote and published the first set of rules in 1743.

In 1867, the Marquess of Queensberry, a British sportsman, introduced rules that saved the sport from a second extinction. The "Queensberry Rules," which include the use of hand strikes only, gloves, three-minute rounds, one-minute rest-periods, and a 10-second recovery period following a knockout, still influence amateur and professional boxing and kickboxing today.

Muay Thai, the national sport of Thailand, is an ancient martial art known originally as Siamese-style boxing. King Naresuan of Siam made Muay Thai a part of military training during his reign from 1590 to 1605. This martial art utilized the arms, legs, knees, and elbows as weapons and proved effective in combat during Siam's fight for independence against Burma. The effectiveness of Muay Thai received more attention in the early 18th century during the reign of King Phra Chao Sua, the Tiger King. Phra Chao Sua was a skilled fighter who would disguise himself as a commoner to enter boxing events and test his fighting skills against local champions. His style of fighting influenced strategies that are still used today. It was Nai Khanom Tom, however, who elevated Muay Thai to legendary proportions. He was a skilled fighter who became a prisoner of war in Burma in the late 18th century. King Mangra of Burma held a festival in Rangoon and selected Nai Kahnom Tom as an opponent for his fighters, who had their own style of boxing. Nai Khanom Tom defeated 10 of the king's best fighters consecutively and gained the admiration of the king. As a result, he was given his freedom.

Until the 1930s, fighters wore no protective equipment and wrapped their hands with hemp rope. If both fighters agreed, the hemp was dipped in glue and rolled in broken pieces of glass. The sport was popularized in the 1920s and, to lessen injury, regular boxing gloves were introduced in the 1930s. Subsequently, bouts were staged in modern boxing rings and the sport became regulated.

Growth

Kickboxing is a cardiovascular workout that uses the hands, feet, knees, and elbows, and mimics kickboxing training to obtain health and fitness benefits. Workouts based on boxing and kickboxing entered the mainstream in the late 1990s and appeal equally to men and women. Today, most health clubs and martial arts schools offer some type of boxing or kickboxing classes. This growth has also been noted by the National Sporting Goods Association. According to their research, 3.0 million people participated in kickboxing in 2003 and another 4.8 million participated in the martial arts.

Benefits

The benefits of exercise are well documented and research continues to support the efficacy of martial arts and kickboxing training as means of improving fitness and health. A 1997 study (Bellinger et al.) found that a 60-minute boxing training session (without kicking) was equivalent in energy expenditure to running about 5.6 mph (9 kph) for 60 minutes on the treadmill. In 1999, the American Council on Exercise (ACE) investigated the physiological effects and benefits of kickboxing (American Council on Exercise, 1999). The researchers found that the activity provides a workout sufficient to improve and maintain cardio-vascular fitness, and noted some additional benefits, such as increased strength and flexi-bility, improved coordination, and sharper reflexes.

Jumping rope may also be an integral part of kickboxing training, and its benefits have been acknowledged in several studies. Jumping rope develops neuromuscular skills, muscular strength, and cardiovascular endurance, and thus is an excellent complement to kickboxing training.

Workout Types and Styles

The purpose of this book is to provide guidelines for conducting both equipment-based and non-equipment-based kickboxing workouts. It must be emphasized that the guidelines presented here are based on the premise that all workouts will be conducted for non-combative purposes.

It is expected, however, that participants in **equipment-based workouts** will naturally experience accidental contact. For example, when teaching defensive drills, you may assign participants to work in pairs, with one throwing slow-speed punches while the other practices **slipping.** Participants may react slowly or move in the wrong direction and occasionally be tapped with a glove on the chin or forehead. Although contact may be slow and controlled, you must still supervise these types of exercises. Participants should never be allowed to perform any sparring. It increases the liability of risk and is clearly outside the scope of practice for a fitness professional.

Equipment-based Workouts

Equipment-based workouts are designed to allow participants to spend a defined amount of time performing kickboxing skills using the heavy bag, punching mitts, kicking pads, speed bags, and/or jump rope, and may be made up of several components. Following a general warm-up, for instance, you may spend 10 to 15 minutes leading participants through basic footwork, punches, kicks, and combinations before moving to performance drills using equipment. The participants may then work together performing the drills for two or three work periods and then be assigned another skill.

Workouts may also be structured as circuits, where stations are set up in a circle or row and participants rotate between pieces of equipment. Stations may include exercises for strength, flexibility, and conditioning. If equipment is limited, arrange for participants to alternate between equipment stations and non-equipment stations or work in pairs.

Non-equipment-based Workouts

Non-equipment-based workouts mirror a traditional aerobics class in that the instructor leads participants through a warm-up and specific boxing and/or kickboxing skills designed to elicit a certain intensity. Movements and combinations are typically based on 32-count phrasing. One punch is typically performed every 2 counts and a kick is usually performed every 2 or 4 counts. Higher-intensity combinations may be performed at a faster tempo of 1 (punches) or 2 counts (punches and/or kicks) for brief work periods.

Exercise

Science

CHAPTER TWO

Safe Participation

Encourage potential participants to observe a class to understand the types of movements that are involved before participating in a kickboxing workout. It is your responsibility to create and maintain a safe environment for all participants regardless of their experience, skill, or level of conditioning. Each participant should be directed to perform any given movement at his or her own pace. Ensure that all participants, especially beginners, are executing each skill and movement properly before increasing intensity or moving on to advanced techniques. Most injuries are simply a result of too much, too soon—a combination of fatigue, poor form, and excessive force.

Equipment maintenance is another issue of safe participation. Because of the wear and tear imposed on equipment, regularly scheduled inspection, maintenance, and replacement should be performed when indicated. A participant without the proper protective equipment (e.g., handwraps or gloves) should not be allowed to participate in equipment-based classes. USA Boxing, the national governing body for Olympic-style boxing, recommends that training equipment utilized by multiple users (e.g., gloves, heavy bags, mats, punch mitts) be cleansed with a solution of water, soap, and 10% household bleach before and after use (USA Boxing, 2000). For purposes of hygiene, hand wraps should be washed after each workout. Talcum powder or foot powder can be sprinkled into the gloves once or twice a week to help absorb sweat and minimize odor.

Frequency

While the physically active participant may be able to participate in a single kickboxing workout with minimal or no soreness, this will not be the case with a new participant. A beginning participant who has not been physically active should participate in kickboxing workouts on non-consecutive days during the first week. This will allow the musculoskeletal system adequate time to adapt to the new stresses of using muscles for different movements and at different angles. The most common complaints of soreness following a kickboxing workout focus on the shoulders, hips, thighs, and calves. Refer participants to an appropriate healthcare practitioner if soreness, aches, or pains persist for more than three days.

With respect to exercise adherence, remember that a negative exercise experience, such as post-exercise soreness or injury, affects a participant's ability to maintain an exercise program. Therefore, you are obligated to create a positive experience for all participants.

Intensity

In some kickboxing workouts, there will be instances when exercises are performed at an anaerobic intensity for short periods of time. Because of this, each participant must pass the "talk test" following an active rest period. (The talk test measures exercise intensity using observation of respiration effort and the ability to talk while exercising.) If needed, the rest period should be extended so that every participant adequately recovers before moving on to the next portion of the class. This is critical because fatigue results in a breakdown in proper form that can easily lead to injury. Also, remind participants to relax when performing any movements or drills. Tense muscles can easily tire out even the most highly conditioned participant.

Time

The duration of a kickboxing workout varies from 45 to 90 minutes. There should be enough time devoted to each segment: warm-up, conditioning, cool-down, flexibility, and strengthening. Unlike amateur and professional kickboxers, participants are not necessarily performing any additional conditioning exercises. Thus, each workout should include an aerobic segment that is 20 minutes or longer.

Type

The availability of equipment, coupled with the skill and experience of the instructor, will determine if the workout is equipment-based, non-equipment-based, or a mixed format that incorporates both types. Instructors who are experienced teaching other types of workouts may be competent enough to teach a non-equipment-based class within a short period of time once they become proficient in basic kickboxing skills. However, this is not the case with equipment-based workouts. Instructors should have quality experience in the martial arts or kickboxing and must be competent in all skills and in using all types of equipment before conducting an equipment-based kickboxing workout.

Aerobic Stimulus

The aerobic stimulus in kickboxing is created through various means, including upper- and lower-extremity movements, a combination of punches and kicks, the speed of the movements, the number of repetitions performed, time between repetitions, and resistance created by the equipment (e.g., weight of the gloves and heavy bags).

Because of the potential to quickly create an anaerobic stimulus, focus on the warm-up and

a gradual progression. Speed combinations, speed kicking, or kicks above waist level should only be performed once participants are warmed up and working within their respective target heart-rate zones.

Kinesiology

All kickboxing movements rely on the sequential coordination of several muscle groups to execute a given punch, kick, or movement. For example, a jab is not simply the result of elbow extension. It is the sequential combination of several actions, including elbow joint extension, shoulder joint flexion, shoulder girdle abduction, trunk flexion and lateral flexion, trunk rotation, knee extension (rear leg), hip extension, and ankle joint plantarflexion. Table 2.1 lists the actions of all extremities required to execute the given punch, kick, or strike to the point of impact from a referenced position (**on-guard position**; see page 25). Note that this table accounts for the significant movements in all variations.

Dynamic Stretching

Dynamic stretching refers to movement-oriented stretching that uses rhythmic actions that are sport-specific. There are two types of dynamic stretching: active and ballistic. Active dynamic stretching usually starts with small movements that increase to larger movements or a wider range of motion. An example of active

Table 2.1

Actions involved in kickboxing punches, kicks, and strikes

Punches	Joint action	Jab	Straight right	Left hook	Uppercut	Elbow strike
Shoulder Joint	Flexion	x	x	x	x	x
Elbow Joint	Extension	x	x		x	
	Flexion			x	x	x
Trunk	Lateral flexion	x			x	x
	Extension				x	
	Rotation	x	x	x	x	x
Hip Joint	Flexion	x	x			
	Extension	x	x		x	x
	Internal rotation		x	x	x	x
Knee Joint	Flexion	x				
	Extension	x	x		x	x
Ankle Joint	Dorsiflexion			x	x	x
	Plantarflexion	x	x	x	x	x
Kicks		**Front**	**Roundhouse**	**Side**	**Rear**	**Knee strike**
Trunk	Lateral flexion		x	x	x	
	Extension	x			x	x
	Flexion				x	
	Rotation		x			x
Hip Joint	Flexion	x	x	x	x	x
	Extension				x	
	External rotation	x	x	x		x
	Internal rotation	x				
	Abduction		x	x		
Knee Joint	Flexion	x	x	x	x	x
	Extension	x	x	x	x	
Ankle Joint	Dorsiflexion	x		x	x	x
	Plantarflexion	x	x			x

dynamic stretching is a warm-up that incorporates **front kicks** at knee level and then gradually progresses to the waist or above the waist. Ballistic dynamic stretching uses rapid bouncing or bobbing motions. An example is a warm-up including footwork drills or shadowboxing while moving around on the balls of the feet. This type of stretching continues to be a topic of controversy for most sports; however, proponents maintain its value for promoting dynamic flexibility, especially in the martial arts.

Both types of dynamic stretching exercises are appropriate for kickboxing because of their warm-up value and rehearsal effect for specific kickboxing skills. Risk of injury can be minimized during ballistic movements by controlling the movements and giving participants an opportunity to adapt prior to increasing the duration or intensity.

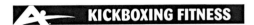

Teaching a Kickboxing Workout

CHAPTER THREE

W hile portions of this chapter and Chapter Four are addressed specifically to group fitness instructors, the information can be applied to one-on-one training as well. It is important for personal trainers to understand effective workout design and proper modifications and progression.

Equipment

Only the highest quality equipment should be used and each piece of equipment should be used solely for its intended purpose. While this may seem like common sense, it must be emphasized that inferior equipment and the misuse of equipment will increase the risk of injury. Supervise the use of all equipment and teach each participant how to use every piece of equipment correctly and safely.

Hand Wraps

The use of hand wraps is a must for all participants and is the first defense against hand injuries. Teach each participant how to properly wrap the hands prior to putting on a pair of gloves (Figure 3.1). Hand wraps that are 2 inches (5.1 cm) wide and at least 150 to 170 inches (3.8 to 4.3 m) long will provide

Figure 3.1
Basic handwrap

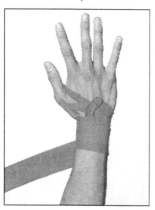

1. Anchor a loop over the thumb and cross wrap diagonally down and across the back of the hand. Wrap snugly twice around the wrist.

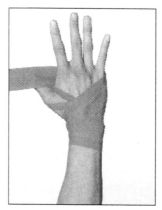

2. Wrap diagonally across the back of the hand and end with the wrap across the palm of the hand.

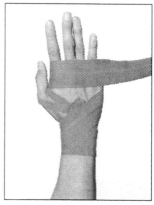

3. Wrap around the knuckles at least two times and end with the wrap across the palm of the hand. The edge of wrap should not be any higher than half way up the first knuckle.

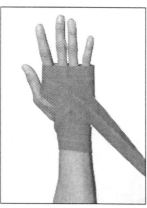

4. Wrap diagonally down and across the back of the hand. Note that this "X" pattern will be repeated in the wrapping.

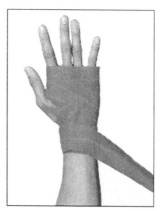

5. Wrap snugly twice around the wrist.

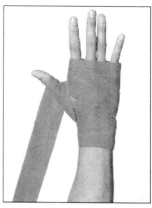

6. Loop around the thumb from front to back.

adequate padding over the knuckles and protection for the wrist joint, fingers, and thumb. The wrist joint must be wrapped securely to minimize movement, and athletic tape may be used under or over the handwraps for extra support. Knuckle guards (½- to ¾-inch thick foam) may be placed on top of the knuckles prior to wrapping for further cushioning and protection.

Figure 3.1
(continued)

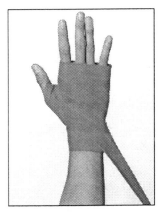

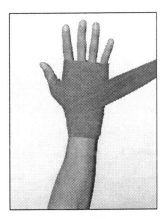

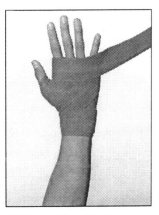

7. Wrap diagonally down and across the back of the hand and at least once across the wrist.

8. Continue the "X" pattern. Wrap up and across back of the hand.

9. Wrap at least twice across the knuckles.

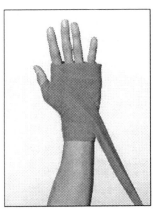

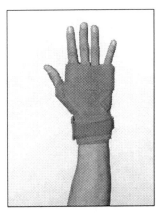

10. Wrap down and across and at least twice around the wrist.

11. Continue the "X" pattern and make sure you have enough wrap left to wrap snugly around the wrists. Note that the finished wrap should be snug and comfortable, but not tight.

Gloves

Gloves should offer maximum protection and be designed for hitting both a heavy bag and punching mitts. Gloves that weigh between 12 and 16 ounces are appropriate for this dual role. Quality gloves are made of leather, offer good support for the wrist, and have attached thumbs (i.e., the thumb is anchored to the glove and cannot move independently) (Figure 3.2). Most glove manufacturers now offer gloves with laces or with elastic/velcro wraps. While manufacturers offer gloves specifically for kickboxing classes, they may not necessarily offer the best protection for the hands. When in doubt, choose the type of gloves used by amateur and professional boxers for training purposes.

Heavy Bags

Most heavy bags found on the market are durable enough to withstand both punching and kicking. Canvas heavy bags are inexpensive and adequate for classes that are conducted several times a week (Figure 3.3). Leather bags are more expensive and can better handle everyday wear and tear. When selecting a heavy bag, be sure that the seams are reinforced and provide a smooth surface for both punching and kicking. Freestanding heavy bags are another inexpensive alternative to hanging heavy bags and are portable. The bases of these bags are usually held down by weights or filled with water or sand for balance (Figure 3.4). One potential drawback to

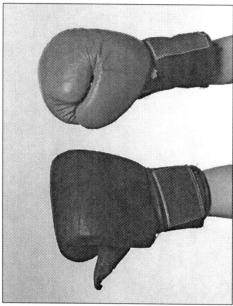

Figure 3.2
The glove on top has an attached thumb, which helps prevent thumb injuries.

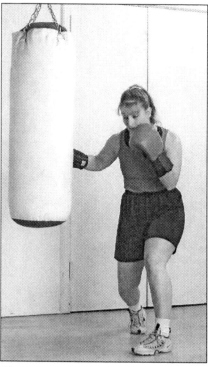

Figure 3.3
Canvas heavy bag

freestanding bags is that there may be some movement upon contact. To minimize the risk of injury, train participants to punch correctly and safely before doing any bagwork.

Punching Mitts

Punching mitts are primarily used to work on basic offense, defense, and conditioning drills. There should be a balance between the weight of the mitt and the protection it provides the user. The mitt should have foam that is thick enough to absorb the shock of the punch and a secure strap or glove on the back to prevent it from sliding off during drills. A qualified instructor or other experienced individual should be holding the punching mitts and provide individualized feedback to the participant on his or her form and mechanics. The proper sequence of punches,

number of repetitions, and placement must be communicated between the mitt holder and participant and, if necessary, the participant should walk through the drill at slow speed. Each punch should be met with a firm tap of the mitt, thereby providing some resistance and minimizing the eccentric loading placed on the arms of the mitt holder (Figure 3.5). To minimize injury to the hand and wrist joint, participants must wear gloves weighing at least 12 to 16 ounces with good padding for the knuckles.

Kicking Pads

Also known as Thai pads, kicking pads are typically two times longer than punching mitts. They cover the forearm and are thicker to absorb the shock of a kick or knee strike. Lighter kicking pads may also be used for punching. When used as a pair, kicking pads create a large

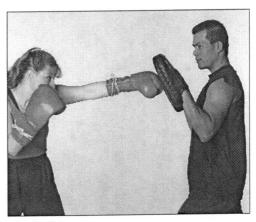

Figure 3.5
When using a punching mitt, meet each punch with some resistance to minimize eccentric loading on the shoulder girdle and joint.

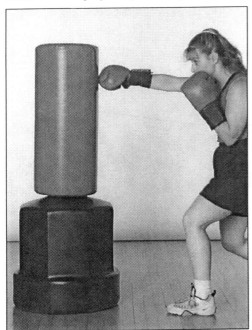

Figure 3.4
Freestanding heavy bag

surface that better absorbs the force of a kick or knee strike (Figure 3.6).

Body Shields

Body shields are designed primarily for absorbing the impact of a kick, but may be used for punching as well. Because of this, select body shields that have the thickest and most dense padding. They should be big enough to provide a large kicking target and also protect the holder.

As with punching mitts, the holder and the participant must communicate and understand the specific kicking and/or punching sequence, number of repetitions, placement, and angle. The participant should first walk through the drill at slow speed. This will help prevent the holder from being inadvertently punched or kicked. To further prevent injury, the holder must position the body shield close to the body and stay light on his or her feet and move with the momentum as needed. Also, the holder must be cautioned to avoid excessive movement since it may cause the participant to hyperextend his or her joints should the body shield suddenly be moved out of range. Therefore, it is paramount that the holder gives full attention to the exercise and allows the participant the opportunity to execute each punch or kick safely (Figure 3.7).

Figure 3.6
Proper use of kicking pads or Thai pads

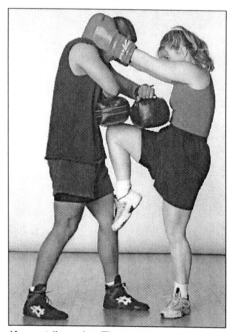

Knee strike using Thai pads

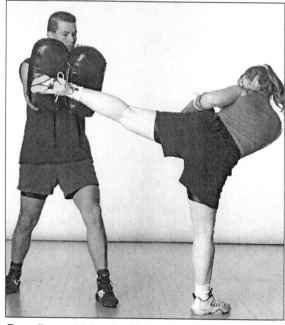

Roundhouse kick using Thai pads

Figure 3.7
Body shield

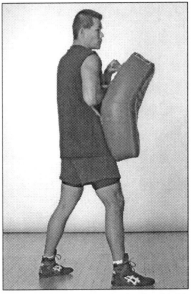

Correct positioning of a body shield

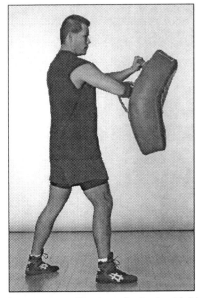

Improper positioning of a body shield

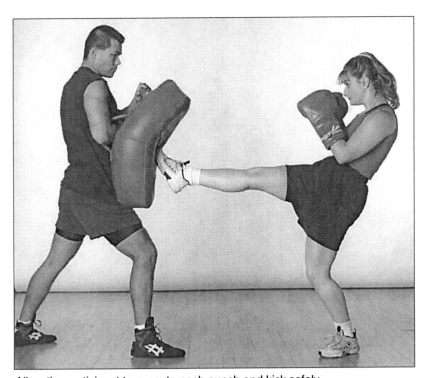

Allow the participant to execute each punch and kick safely.

Speed Bags

Speed bags may not be practical for all kickboxing workouts; if you decide to use them, consider the size of the speed bag, the type of swivel mechanism, and the platform. Larger speed bags are ideal for novice participants, since they are slower than smaller speed bags. Swivel mechanisms are designed either for speed or to make it easy to change the size of the speed bag. Speed bag platforms must be sturdy and stable enough to minimize vibration and be adjustable in height. Participants must wear hand wraps when striking the speed bag (Figure 3.8).

Jump Ropes

Most jump ropes on the market today are appropriate for a kickboxing class. Better quality jump ropes are designed for speed and are made of either leather or plastic. Provide jump ropes of different lengths to accommodate all participants. To determine if a jump rope is the right length,

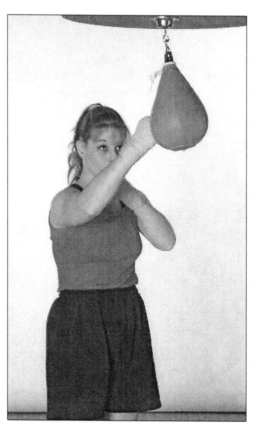

Figure 3.8
Adjust the height of the speed bag so that the striking surface (round center) is at approximately eye level.

stand on the middle of the rope with your feet together and pull the handles in front of you toward your shoulders. The handles should come up to your armpits but not past your shoulders (Figure 3.9). A wooden floor is ideal for jumping rope because it is smooth and offers minimal resistance to the rope.

Limit jumping rope to 30-second intervals for novice participants and gradually increase the time. Encourage participants to be patient because it is a learned skill. Remind them to turn the rope only with their wrists, keep their upper arms close to the body with their forearms at approximately a 45-degree angle toward the floor, and jump only as high as needed to allow the jump rope to pass underneath. Relax the shoulders and land on the balls of the feet (Figure 3.10).

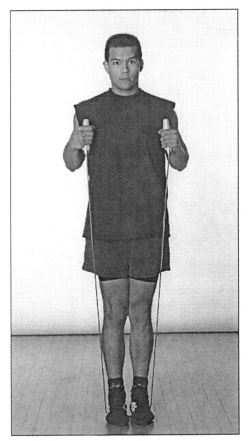

Figure 3.9
The handles of a jump rope should come up to the armpits but not past the shoulders.

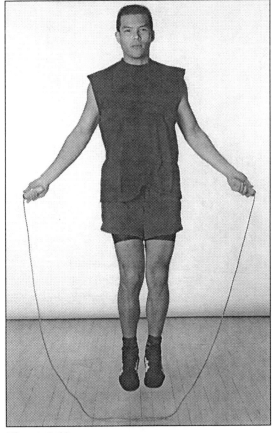

Figure 3.10
Proper jump-rope form, with the forearms at approximately a 45-degree angle toward the floor.

Basic Jump Rope Variations

To ease transitions between variations, insert a single bounce.

Single Bounce—Jump once in each rotation of the rope.
Double Bounce—Jump twice in each rotation of the rope.

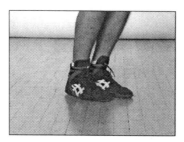 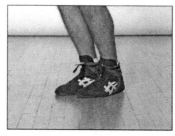

Figure 3.11 Skier—Jump side to side like you are skiing.

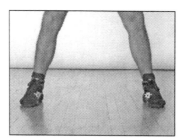 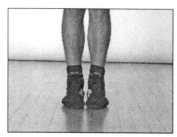

Figure 3.12 Side Straddle—Perform a jumping jack using only your feet.

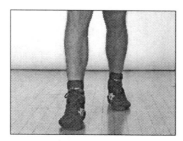 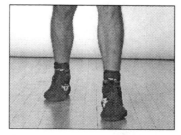

Figure 3.13 Front Straddle—Jump with one foot in front and the other in back, switching the positions of your feet with each jump.

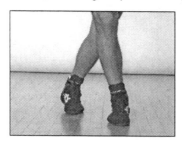 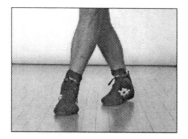

Figure 3.14 Cross Step—During the first rotation of the rope, jump with your feet spread apart; on the second, jump and cross your legs.

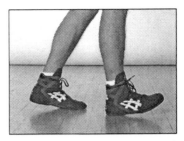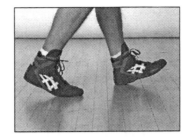

Figure 3.15 Heel Exchange—Jump and touch one heel to the ground in front of you, switching heels with each jump.

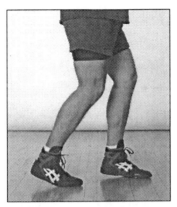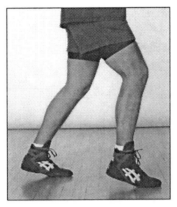

Figure 3.16 Toe Exchange—Jump and touch one toe to the ground behind you, switching feet with each jump.

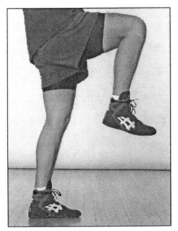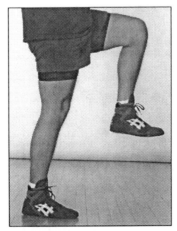

Figure 3.17 Jogging Step—Turn the rope and imitate jogging in place by stepping over it and switching feet with each jump.

Attire

Participants should wear comfortable workout attire and remove all jewelry prior to the workout. This includes necklaces, earrings, watches, or anything that might become caught on equipment or on another participant during class. High-top cross-training shoes are recommended because they provide adequate cushion, lateral support, and stability for the ankle joint during jump rope exercises and may protect the feet in the event that improper contact is made during kicking. Regardless of the type of shoe, the sole should have a smooth surface to allow pivoting with little resistance.

Environment

The biggest consideration in any group fitness class is space; this is especially true for a kickboxing class because of the potential for accidental contact between participants. Non-equipment-based classes should have no more than 25 participants per instructor. In equipment-based classes, the ideal class size is no more than 18 participants per instructor, thereby enabling you to work with no more than nine pairs of participants. Regardless of the type of class, offer continual cueing and immediately provide corrective feedback when movements are performed incorrectly. The *ACSM Health/Fitness Facility Standards and Guidelines* recommends that the workout room have mirrors on two of the four walls and room temperature be maintained at 66 to 70°F (18 to 21°C) (American College of Sports Medicine, 1997).

Music

Non-equipment-based kickboxing workouts that are choreographed to music should be at an appropriate tempo to allow even the least-coordinated participant to complete and execute a given movement and combination without difficulty. Music tempos of 100 beats per minute (bpm) are appropriate for warm-up and cool-down, and tempos between 120 and 128 bpm are appropriate for the conditioning portion of the class. Note that tempos higher than 128 bpm place participants at greater risk for injury since proper form and mechanics may be sacrificed for speed. In addition, sound levels should not exceed 85 decibels.

Modifications

You are obligated to provide modifications and/or alternatives to every kickboxing drill when indicated, especially to participants who may have injuries. For example, to provide a lower-intensity workout, emphasize punches, footwork, and shadowboxing. Kicks may also be performed less frequently and no higher than waist level. Emphasize linear kicks over movements that are more complex and require more coordination. For example, individuals having coordination problems when jumping rope may wish to consider mimicking the jump rope movement without the rope until they become more comfortable with their footwork.

Class Introduction/Health Screening

Because kickboxing has the potential to be a vigorous and high-intensity activity, each participant must be properly screened and receive medical clearance prior to participation. The American College of Sports Medicine recommends that males 45 years of age or older and women 55 years of age or older receive medical clearance along with a graded exercise testing prior to participating in vigorous activity (American College of Sports Medicine, 2000). Whether or not you are responsible for performing the screening, communicate with all participants at the beginning of each class and inquire about any new health conditions or injuries that

might be exacerbated with the planned kickboxing workout. Provide modifications accordingly.

Cueing

Continuous cueing is essential for a smooth workout. In non-equipment-based classes, provide cues several measures or beats prior to the movement. This also helps provide smooth transitions between movements. Encourage participants to watch themselves in the mirror and pay careful attention to their form and mechanics. Monitor all participants closely and immediately provide corrective feedback when needed.

Intensity Monitoring

Monitor exercise intensity via heart rate, rating of perceived exertion, or the talk test where appropriate. Most importantly, encourage participants to pace themselves and maintain a level of intensity that is comfortable, yet challenging.

Programming

Components

Kickboxing workouts are made up of several components and corresponding skills. The skills listed here are provided as examples and not all components are necessarily performed in a given workout. Please note these components are not listed in any particular order.

1. Upper-body skills (jabs, straight rights, uppercuts, hooks, elbow strikes)
2. Lower-body skills (front kicks, side kicks, roundhouse kicks, rear kicks, knee strikes)
3. Combinations (upper- and lower-body drills)
4. Conditioning drills (push-ups, curl-ups, jumping rope, jumping jacks)
5. Footwork and defensive drills (ducking, bobbing and weaving, catching, slipping, shuffling)

Note that this book functions as a resource for fitness professionals and is not intended to provide complete or thorough instruction on how to design and instruct a kickboxing workout. Instructors should receive quality instruction, participate in kickboxing seminars, and work with other fitness professionals and martial artists as indicated. The potential types of formats are endless, and are dictated by the creativity and, more importantly, the experience of the instructor.

Warm-up through Cool-down

Below are samples of equipment-based and non-equipment-based workouts and their specific components.

Equipment-based kickboxing workout (sample)

Class warm-up (10–15 minutes)
- Calisthenics
- Dynamic stretching
- Shadowboxing
- Static stretching

Circuit stations (1–3 minute circuits with 30-second active rest periods)
- Jumping rope
- Heavy bag (punching and elbow strikes only)
- Mitt work
- Heavy bag (kicking and kneeing only)
- Push-ups and crunches
- Defensive drills, footwork drills
- Heavy bag (punching and kicking)
- Shadow-kickboxing

- Cool-down and stretching (5–10 minutes)

Non-equipment-based kickboxing workout (sample)

General and specific warm-up (5–10 minutes)
- Marching in place
- Squats
- Bobbing and weaving
- Footwork movements
- Jabs (right and left)
- Straight rights (and straight lefts)
- Hooks (right and left)
- Uppercuts (right and left)
- Elbow strikes (right and left)
- Forearm blocks (right and left)
- Parrying (right and left)
- Knee strikes (right and left)
- Kicks (right and left)
- Stretching major muscle groups
- Conditioning (5 minutes)

Combinations using various punches and strikes

Note: Build the combination from the first punch, then add the second, and so on.

For example:

1st Combination: Left Jab, Straight Right, Left Hook, Right Uppercut

2nd Combination: Straight Right, Hook to the Body, Hook to the Chin, Right Uppercut

- Switch to southpaw stance and repeat
- Conditioning (5 minutes)

Combinations using various kicks and strikes

> **Note:** Build the combination from the first strike, then add the second, and so on.
>
> For example:
>
> *1st Combination:* Front Kick, Side Kick, Back Kick (knee level, then waist level)
>
> *2nd Combination:* Roundhouse Kick, Front Kick, Side Kick (step through with each kick and perform with alternate leg)
>
> • Switch to the other side and repeat
>
> • Water break / Intensity check
>
> • Conditioning (5 minutes)

Combinations using various punches, kicks, and strikes

> **Note:** Build the combination from the first strike, then add the second, and so on.
>
> For example:
>
> *1st Combination:* Left Jab, Straight Right, Front Kick, Left Knee
>
> *2nd Combination:* Left Elbow, Straight Right, Roundhouse Kick
>
> • Defensive drills (ducking, bobbing and weaving, slipping)
>
> • Conditioning (5 minutes)

Jump rope and variations

> • Cool-down (5 minutes)
>
> • Repeat drills used for specific warm-up

Floor work and stretching (15 minutes)

Techniques

K ickboxing movements require fine motor skills and it may take months to years for some participants to coordinate these movements. Because of this, constantly provide instruction and cues to reinforce correct positioning, footwork, offensive skills, and defensive skills.

Positioning

Basic Stance

The boxer's stance permits the greatest possibilities for both offense and defense. The feet should be 1¼- to 1½-times shoulder width and the knees must be flexed at all times. This provides a spring in the legs that makes all forward, lateral, and backward movement easier to execute (Figure 4.1).

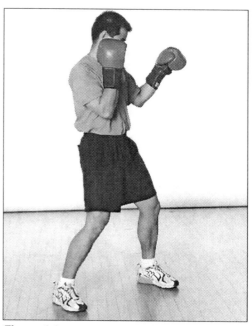

Figure 4.1
Basic stance

For a right-handed individual, the left foot is in front and right foot in back. In this position, the right-hander throws the jab with the left hand. This is known as an **orthodox stance** and will be the reference stance for all movements presented in this book. Conversely, a left-handed individual uses a **southpaw stance** with the right foot in front and left foot in back. The jab is thrown with the right hand.

Foot Alignment

To determine proper foot position, imagine that the front foot is the center point of a clock. The right foot should be somewhere between four and five o'clock (Figure 4.2). Conversely, a southpaw will have the left foot positioned somewhere between seven and eight o'clock.

In an orthodox stance, the feet should be parallel and pointing between one and two o'clock. Conversely, a southpaw should have the feet pointing between ten and eleven o'clock.

Hand Positioning (On-guard position)

In an orthodox stance, the left shoulder is pointing toward the target or opponent and is level with the right. The right hand is positioned between the cheekbone and eyebrow, covering the outer right side of the chin, with the elbow relaxed against the outer right side of the ribs and the palm turned inward, facing the body. The left hand is also positioned between cheekbone and eyebrow level, but is slightly extended from the body by opening up the elbow joint to approximately 90 degrees. The left palm faces away from the body, and the wrist joint maintains a neutral position. Also, the chin is tucked in close to the clavicle. The cue "hands-up" serves as a reminder to participants to maintain the on-guard position (Figure 4.3).

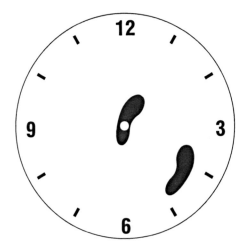

Figure 4.2
Proper foot alignment for the orthodox stance

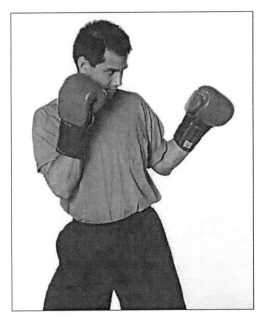

Figure 4.3
The on-guard position

Offense

Striking Surface for Punching

The striking surfaces for all punches should be concentrated primarily on the first two knuckles (the proximal phalanges of the first two digits) (Figure 4.4). To minimize injury, keep the wrist in neutral position as the two knuckles make contact with the target (Figures 4.5). The wrist should not have any flexion or extension (Figure 4.6).

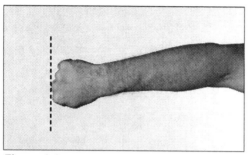

Figure 4.4
Proper striking surface for punching

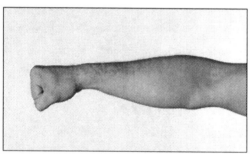

Figure 4.5
Neutral wrist position

Figure 4.6
Improper wrist alignment

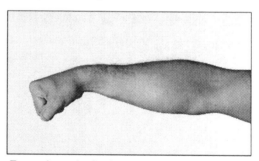

Excessive wrist flexion

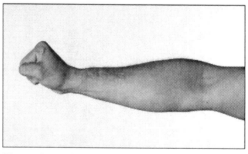

Excessive wrist extension

The Jab

The **jab** keeps opponents off balance, sets up other punches, and can be used for both offense and defense. When a jab is thrown correctly, feet and hands movements are coordinated.

The rear leg pushes through plantarflexion, and knee and hip extension in an explosive manner to close the distance between the participant and the target. The distance between the front and rear foot is temporarily increased during the push-off phase and returns to the regular distance once the ground is covered. Note that the distance between the feet is never decreased at any time. The distance between the feet should be maintained at 1¼- to 1½-times the width of the shoulders with the knees flexed at the start and end of the push-off phase. This footwork is known as the boxer's shuffle and is a fundamental kickboxing skill (Figure 4.7).

The jab is executed through sequential actions during the push-off phase. As the elbow joint extends, the resulting flexion of the shoulder covers the chin (Figure 4.8). There should be no "winding-up," or cocking the hand back, before throwing the jab. The jab should be thrown directly from shoulder-level and retracted immediately once extension or contact is made. The jab can generate power if the entire weight of the body is behind the punch.

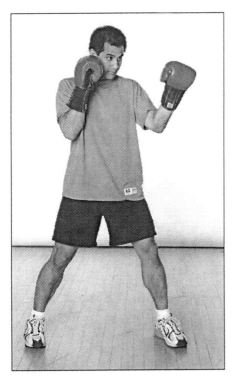

Figure 4.7
Boxer's shuffle

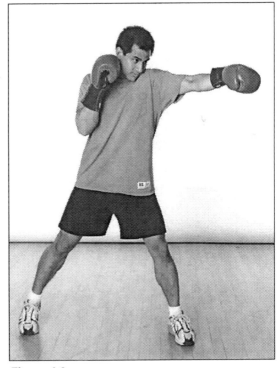

Figure 4.8
Left jab

Straight Right

The **straight right** is usually thrown following the jab but is sometimes thrown as a lead punch. From the on-guard position, the right hand is thrown straight to the target while simultaneously rotating the hip and flexing the shoulder for maximum reach and power. The wrist maintains a neutral position, neither flexed nor extended. The power of this punch is derived from the leverage generated by the simultaneous action of the right leg. The right foot pivots (internal rotation) and pushes off (plantarflexion) when the right hand extends toward the target.

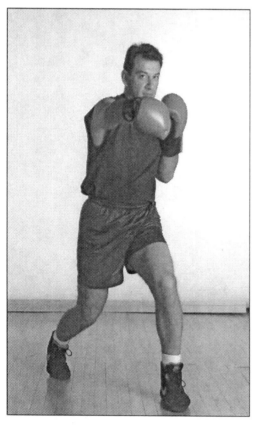

Figure 4.9
Straight right

As in the jab, the resulting flexion of the anterior deltoid covers the chin while the elbow joint maintains a slight bend (Figure 4.9). Once the right is thrown, immediately return to the on-guard position.

Left Hook

The **left hook** is a short-range punch that can be thrown with speed and/or power. A tremendous amount of power may be generated if the entire weight of the body is behind the punch. This punch usually follows a jab or straight right, but may also be used as a lead punch.

The left hook is thrown by bringing the elbow to a horizontal position in line with the same hand, so that the forearm is parallel to the floor. The palm is turned inward, facing the body, and the elbow joint is slightly flexed to approximately 90 degrees. If a hook is being thrown to the body, the hand drops down to the level of the elbow joint.

From the on-guard position, the hook begins with the elbow opening up to 90 degrees as the left shoulder, hip, and ankle rotate in unison by pivoting on both feet (primarily internal rotation of the left foot). The left hand is whipped in an arc toward the target. There should be adequate rotation so that the body hooks the left hand just past the centerline of the body. The right hand maintains its on-guard position while the left hook is executed (Figure 4.10).

Uppercut

The **uppercut** is another short-range punch that is thrown inside, typically targeting the

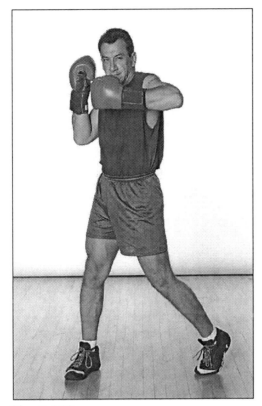

Figure 4.10
Left hook

executed properly, the elbow will maintain a flexed position and remain close to the body. As contact is made with the target, the right hip is driven forward, the right knee joint extends, and both feet pivot (primarily internal rotation of the right foot) to provide more leverage (Figure 4.11). Upon contact, the right hand is immediately returned to the on-guard position.

An uppercut can also be thrown with the left hand (lead hand). From the on-guard position, the knees flex slightly as the left shoulder dips slightly in front. The left hand then extends upward toward the target as the left knee extends and both feet pivot (primarily internal rotation of the left foot). Note that the combined movement

chin. It is usually thrown as a power punch with the right hand following a jab or left hook, and sometimes as a lead punch. Most of the power generated from the uppercut comes from the explosive extension of the trunk, hip, and knee joint.

From the on-guard position, the right hand travels in a short downward arc from its on-guard position on the right side of the chin. The shoulder drops slightly and the hands dip just below the sternum. The hand and shoulder then continue on an upward arc and extend toward the target or chin directly in front. The palm is turned inward, facing the body. If the uppercut is

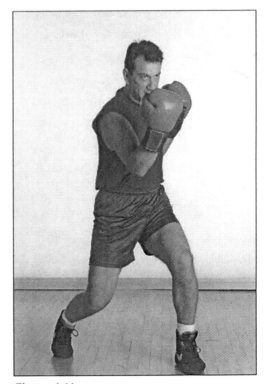

Figure 4.11
Uppercut

of the knee and foot is what generates power for the left uppercut.

Elbow Strikes

In Muay Thai, the point of the elbow is used to strike the opponent from various angles and positions. Elbow strikes are best suited for non-equipment-based workouts due to the high risk of trauma. If elbow strikes are to be incorporated into an equipment-based workout, horizontal elbow strikes should be used.

If an elbow strike is performed on a heavy bag or body shield, contact should not be made with the point of the elbow (the olecranon process), but rather the flat underside surface of the forearm (radial surface of the forearm proximal to the elbow) for a target in front or with the area of the triceps proximal to the elbow for a target to the side or behind the participant.

The body mechanics used for a horizontal elbow strike for a target in front are similar to those used in other punches. If the lead elbow (left elbow) is used, the body mechanics are the same as a left hook; the body and elbow rotate in unison. If the rear elbow (right elbow) is used, the body mechanics are the same as that of the straight right. The elbow should be in a fully flexed position to minimize trauma to the joint. Note that the non-striking hand maintains the on-guard position by covering the chin.

Basic Combinations

An effective kickboxing workout does not require complex punching and/or kicking combinations. The most effective workouts can utilize the simplest combinations as long as they flow naturally from one position to the next. Consider the biomechanics of each movement and ensure that even the least coordinated participant can successfully execute the combination. A stable base is the key to performing all kickboxing movements. Teach participants how to extend their punches without terminal extension to the joints and without losing their balance.

Basic Punching Combinations

1. Double or triple left jab to the chin
2. Left jab to the chin, left jab to the body
3. Left jab to the body, left jab to the chin
4. Left jab to the chin, straight right to the chin (the old one-two)
5. Left jab to the chin, straight right to the body
6. Left jab to the body, straight right to the chin
7. Left jab to chin, straight right to the chin, left hook to the chin
8. Left jab to the body, straight right to the body
9. Left jab to the chin, left hook to the chin
10. Left jab to the chin, straight right to the body, left hook to the chin
11. Straight right to the body, left hook to the chin
12. Straight right to the chin, left hook to the chin
13. Straight right to the chin, left hook to the body

Reprinted with permission from Brown, J. *Ringside Boxing Manual*. Ringside, Inc.

Beginning participants may have an easier time alternating punches with their right and left sides instead of punching with the same hand.

Defense

Catching

Catching is for defense against a left jab. The right glove catches the jab, similar to catching a baseball with a catcher's mitt. As the jab is thrown, the open hand of the defender's right glove meets it with some resistance so that the participant is not hit with his or her own glove. The key to catching a jab is to let it come to you and not reach out to meet it half way. Regardless if one is catching with one or both gloves, the hands must remain at the cheekbone level. If done properly, the jab will be caught directly in front of the participant's face or body (Figure 4.12).

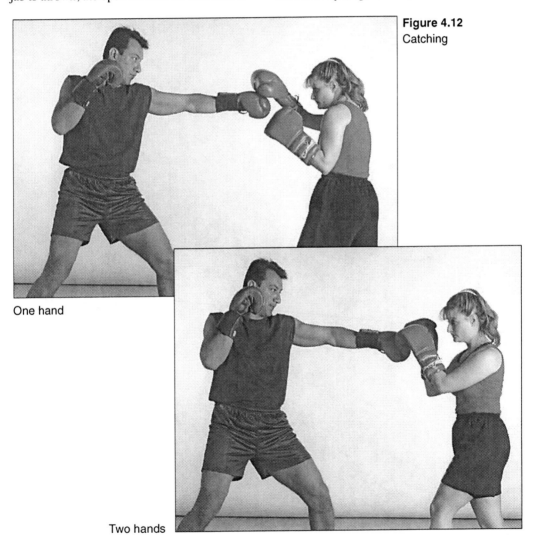

Figure 4.12
Catching

One hand

Two hands

Slipping (inside & outside)

Slipping is a defensive technique used to avoid a punch without moving out of range. To slip a left jab on the outside, the participant laterally flexes the trunk to the right to allow the punch to slip past the left shoulder, and does the opposite to slip a straight right on the inside (Figure 4.13). Note that slipping is primarily a side-to-side movement without any extension of the trunk.

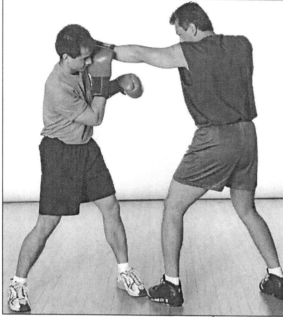

Outside slip

Figure 4.13
Slipping

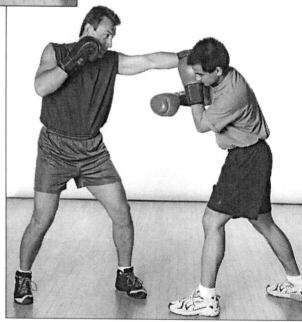

Inside slip

Ducking

Ducking serves to avoid punches while remaining in range for a counterattack. From the on-guard position, the knees flex and the trunk flexes 30 to 45 degrees to either the right or the left relative to the direction of the oncoming punch. There is just enough movement to get out of range from the punch while eye contact is maintained with the target or opponent (Figure 4.14). After ducking, the on-guard position is resumed.

Figure 4.14
Ducking is primarily flexion of the trunk and knee.

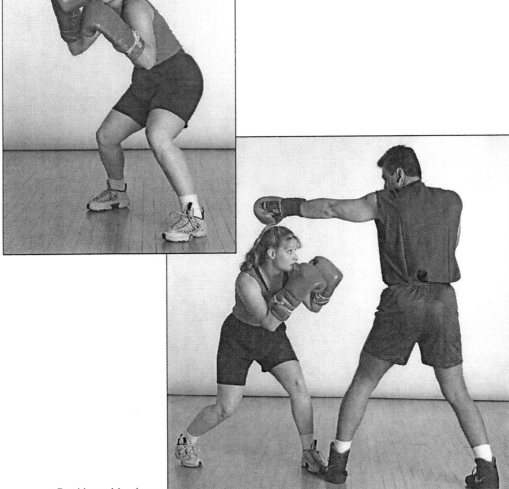

Ducking, side view

Parrying

Unlike catching, **parrying** serves to deflect a punch. Parrying is a subtle movement analogous to a quick, short block (Figure 4.15). This is done to create openings for counterpunches. As with catching, the hands should never reach out, but instead meet the punch close to the body. As the open glove of the right hand meets the jab, it parries the jab to the left by brushing the right hand across the body with just enough movement to deflect the punch out of range. As the right hand parries, the upper body and head move to the right for added defense in case the parry is ineffective or late.

Figure 4.15
Parrying

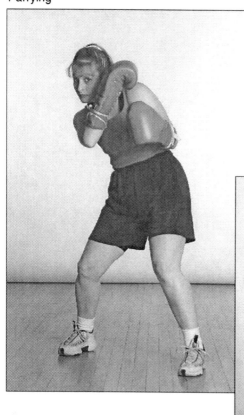
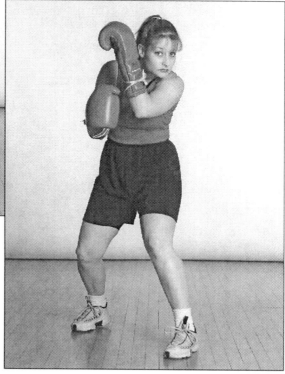

Forearm Block

The forearm block defends against the left hook, **roundhouse kick,** or any other offensive strike that is directed toward the side of the chin or head. As the left hook is initiated, the right hand is raised slightly to cover the chin with the forearm and the body is turned to the left to roll with the punch. The trunk also flexes forward so that the body is inside the arc of the punch (Figure 4.16).

Figure 4.16
Forearm block

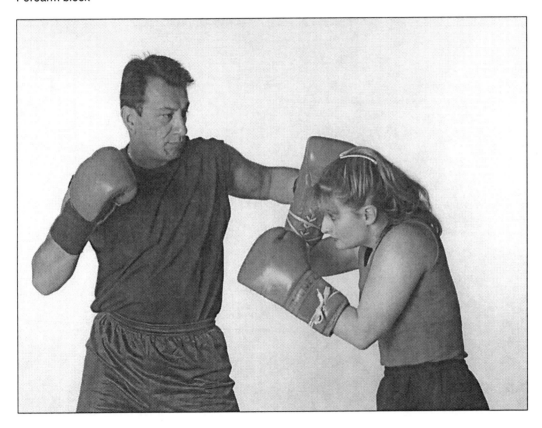

Bob and Weave

Bobbing and weaving is a defensive movement that combines slipping and half-squats to evade a series of punches. From the on-guard position, the front foot (left) takes a small step to the left while the knee joints flex, resulting in a half-squat. There is just enough knee flexion to allow the head to bob under the punch (Figure 4.17). The on-guard position is resumed as the head bobs up and the rear foot resumes its original position and distance from the front leg. The bob and weave can then be initiated on the right side by taking a small step with the rear foot and repeating the above sequence.

Figure 4.17
Bobbing and weaving

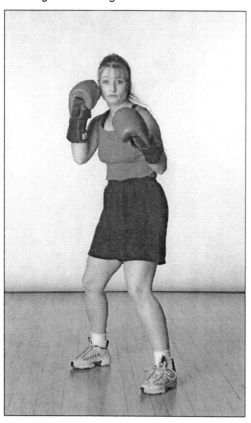

Bobbing and weaving begins
in the on-guard position.

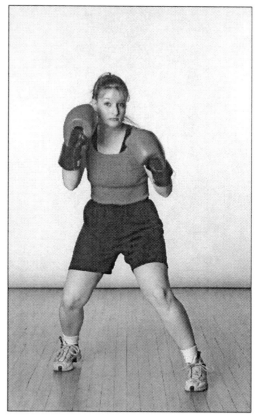

Bobbing and weaving
first to the right

Figure 4.17 (continued)

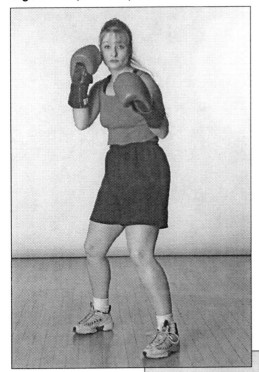

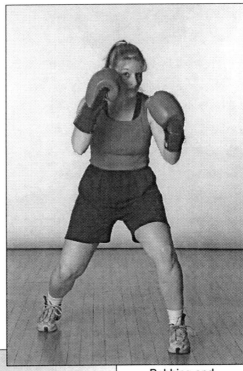

Return to on-
guard position

Bobbing and
weaving to the left

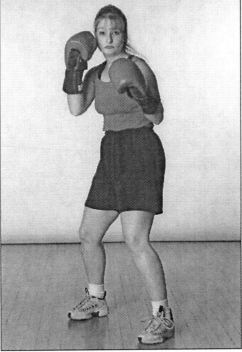

Return to on-guard position

Kicking Techniques

Of all kickboxing skills, kicking is the most difficult to become proficient at because it requires the right combination of conditioning, flexibility, balance, and **proprioception.** The kicks presented here are basic in nature and referenced from a static on-guard position. Proper form and mechanics are musts because of the potential for injury to the lower extremity. For example, a great amount of shear force is placed on the knee if the stationary or support foot fails to pivot simultaneously during a roundhouse kick and puts the anterior cruciate ligament at risk. Likewise, there is risk to the hip joint and iliotibial band should internal rotation occur during a front kick. With any type of kick, participants must maintain a slight bend in the knee joint and be cautioned against hyperextension. These risks underscore the importance of teaching kicking safely and correctly before progressing to advanced kicks.

To minimize the risk of injury, kicks should be performed as part of an active warm-up or following the warm-up, be well below the end-limit of a participant's range of motion, and be executed without any power. Flexibility exercises for the lower extremity following the warm-up may also minimize the risk of injury. The target for all kicks is directly in front of the participant unless referenced otherwise.

Front Kick

Rear Leg. The **front kick** is the easiest kick to learn, as it is primarily a linear movement.

From the on-guard position, the rear leg (right leg) is brought into flexion at both the hip joint and the knee joint. The ankle is dorsiflexed and the foot is positioned directly under the knee as the toes are extended and curled toward you. The foot of the support leg must externally rotate slightly as the hip and knee joints are flexed (Figure 4.18).

Figure 4.18
Front kick, rear leg

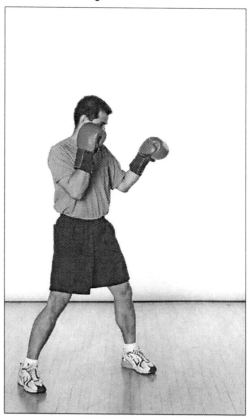

Ready position

To execute the front kick, the knee joint is extended as the ball of the foot (with the toes curled back) or the heel makes contact with the target. As the knee joint extends, the trunk also extends, which serves as a counterbalance and increases the reach of the kick. Note that the kicking motion is similar to a leg press motion. To further minimize the shear forces on the knee joint, the support leg (left) is kept slightly flexed and the foot continues to pivot (external rotation) as the kick extends (Figure 4.19). As soon as the kick is executed or contact is made with equipment, the leg is retracted (reverse order of execution of the kick) and the on-guard position is resumed.

Figure 4.19
Front kick, rear leg, execution

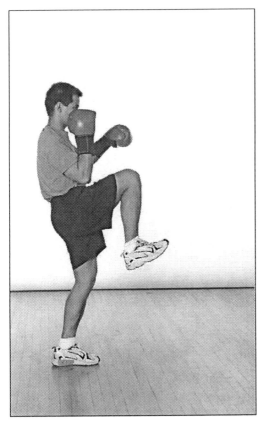

Preparation

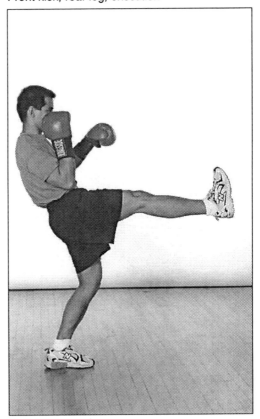

Front Leg. The preparation and execution of this kick with the front leg is the same as the rear leg (Figure 4.20). Performed with the front leg, this kick will not produce as much force since there is a biomechanical disadvantage compared to the rear leg.

Variation

Another variation of the front kick performed by the rear leg is to first align the front foot (support leg) in a neutral position by taking a small step or positioning the foot so that the toes and both hips point directly at the target (twelve noon) (Figure 4.21). This is done prior to the preparatory phase of the front kick. This variation is ideal when performing these kicks on a thick carpeted surface where pivoting may be difficult or for participants who have problems coordinating the pivoting movements on the balls of their feet. In these instances front kicks should be performed with the rear leg only.

Figure 4.20
Front kick, front leg

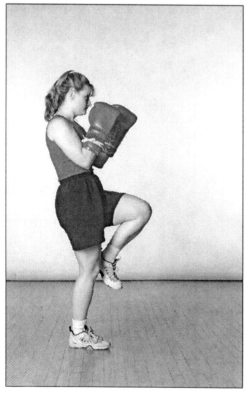

Preparation

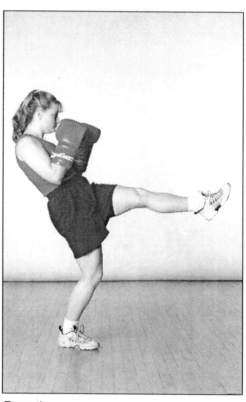

Execution

Figure 4.21
Variation for front kick

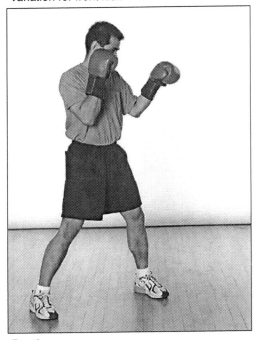

Ready

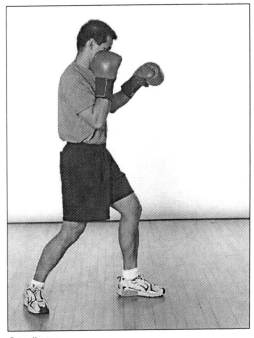

Small step

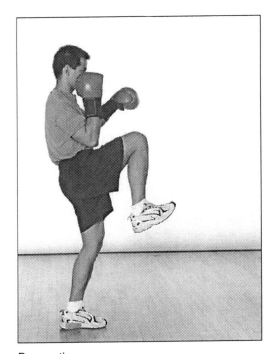

Preparation

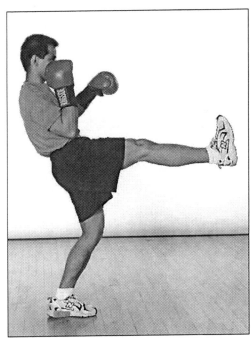

Execution

Side Kick

The **side kick** is best executed from an orthodox stance using the front leg or from a modified on-guard position with the feet aligned next to each other and shoulder-width apart.

Front Leg. The hip and knee joints of the front leg are brought into flexion and the foot is directly under the knee with the toes extended and pulled toward you. There is some pivoting (external rotation) of the

Figure 4.22
Side kick, front leg only

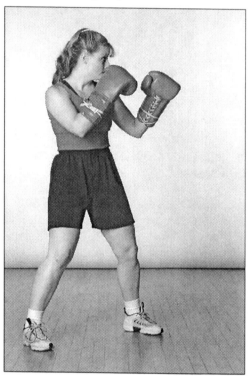

Ready position

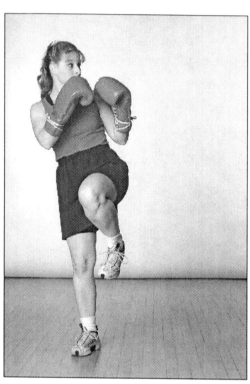

Preparation

support foot that occurs in this preparation phase (Figure 4.22). As the kick is extended, the support foot continues to pivot (external rotation). For safety, there should be enough pivoting (at least 45 degrees) so that the toe of the support foot is pointing opposite the target (i.e., the heel is pointing in the direction of the target). Contact is made with the heel, lateral side of the foot, or plantar surface of the foot (Figure 4.23).

Figure 4.23
Side kick, execution

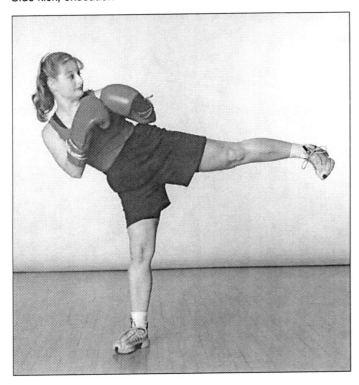

Variation

Another variation is to take a small step or position the foot of the support leg to point at four o'clock (or eight o'clock from a southpaw stance) relative to the target (twelve noon) (Figure 4.24). This is done prior to the preparatory phase of the side kick. This variation is ideal for participants who have problems coordinating the pivoting movements on the balls of their feet and when performing these kicks on a thick carpeted surface where pivoting may be difficult.

Figure 4.24
Variation for side kick

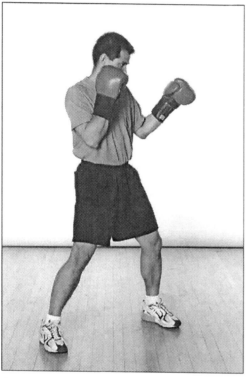

Ready

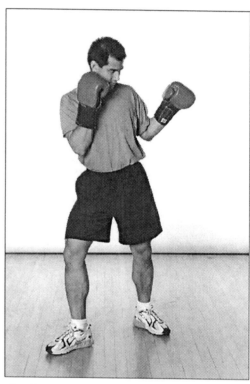

Small step

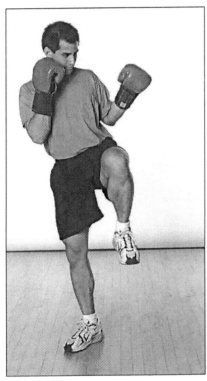

Ready

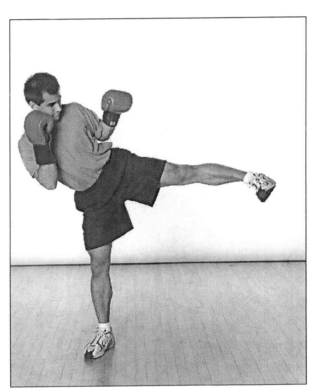

Execution

Roundhouse Kick (Wheel Kick)

Rear leg. The **roundhouse kick** can generate a tremendous amount of power, which is dictated by the leg used (front or rear), leg speed, and flexibility. The preparation for the rear leg is somewhat similar to that of the front kick. While there is flexion of the knee and hip joints, there is also abduction of the hip joint that is continuous from the beginning of the kick until contact is made (circular translation) (Figure 4.25). This

Figure 4.25
Roundhouse kick, rear leg

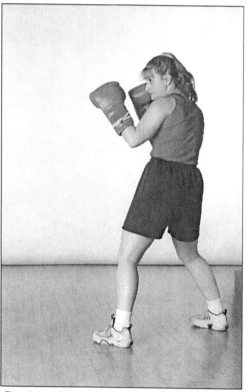

Ready position

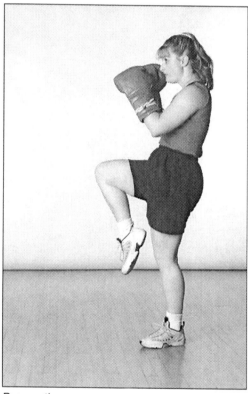

Preparation

kick relies on timing to minimize injury. The kick must be executed so that the support foot pivots (externally rotates) as the kicking leg simultaneously begins its travel toward the target.

Contact should be made with the instep of the foot (articulation of the tarsal and tibia) with the ankle joint in plantarflexion, or with the lower leg (tibia) (Figure 4.26).

Figure 4.26
Roundhouse kick, rear leg; execution

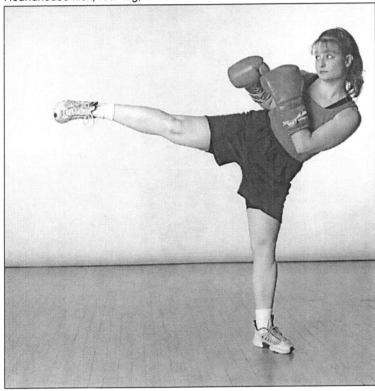

Front leg. The mechanics for a roundhouse kick performed with the front leg are the same as the rear leg, but the amount of travel needed to bring the knee joint into flexion and the hip joint into flexion and adduction is minimal. Again, the kick must be executed so that the support foot pivots (externally rotates) as the front leg simultaneously moves toward the target (Figure 4.27).

Figure 4.27
Roundhouse kick, front leg

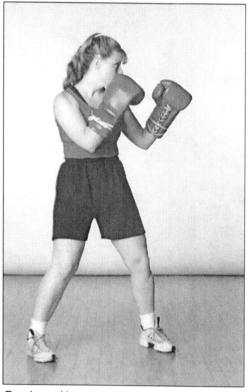

Ready position

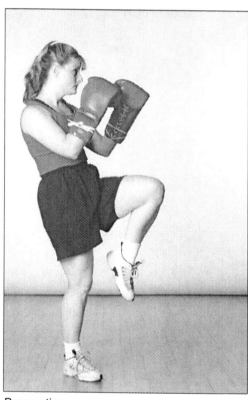

Preparation

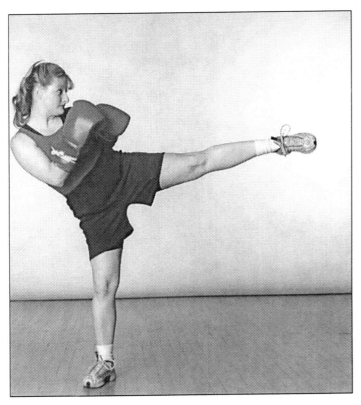

Execution

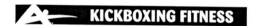

Another variation for performing a roundhouse with the rear leg is to first take a small step with the left foot (support leg) or position the foot so that it is pointing at ten o'clock relative to the target (twelve noon). Using the front leg, the right foot (support leg) steps out or is positioned so that

Figure 4.28
Variation for roundhouse kick, rear leg

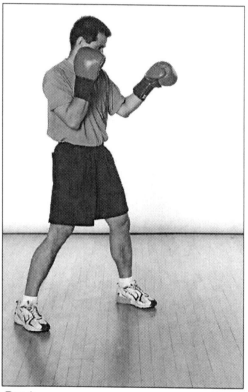

Ready

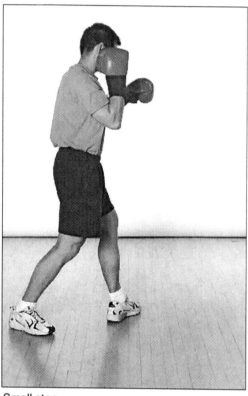

Small step

it is pointing at three o'clock relative to the target. This is done prior to the preparatory phase of the roundhouse (Figure 4.28). This step variation is ideal for participants who have problems coordinating the pivoting movements on the balls of their feet and when performing these kicks on a thick carpeted surface where pivoting may be difficult.

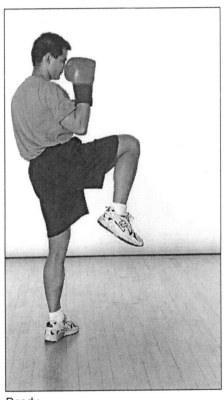

Ready

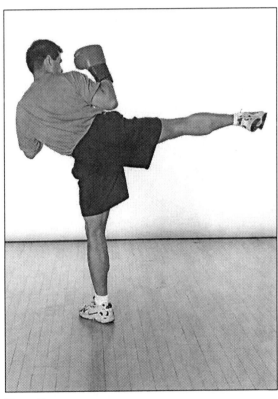

Execution

Rear Kick

Also known as a heel or back kick, the **rear kick** is a primarily linear movement and is easily taught from a standing position with the feet together. More power can be generated from the front leg (left leg) when this kick is executed from the on-guard position. This kick should be performed well below the participant's end range of motion to minimize stresses on the spine.

Front leg. As the head and trunk pivot to sight the target over the left shoulder, both hips and feet also pivot to the left so that both feet are pointing at twelve o'clock. The left knee and hip are then brought into flexion (Figure 4.29) and

Figure 4.29
Rear kick, front leg

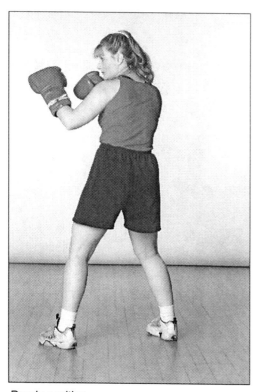

Ready position

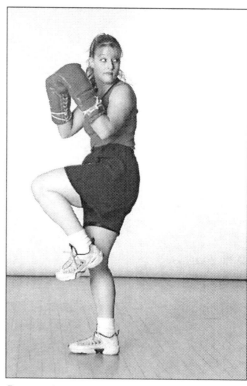

Preparation

the kick is executed by extending the leg through hip extension toward the target. The toes should be pointed toward the floor and impact made primarily with the heel (Figure 4.30). The support leg again maintains a slight bend at the knee as the kick is executed.

Figure 4.30
Rear kick, front leg; execution

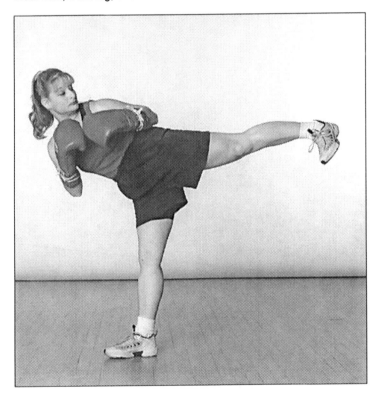

Rear leg. The mechanics when using the rear leg are similar to those of the front leg rear kick. Since the body is already turned to the right, only the head needs to rotate to sight the target over the right shoulder (Figure 4.31). As the kick is executed, the support leg (left) pivots (externally rotates) and maintains a slight bend at the knee (Figure 4.32).

Figure 4.31
Rear kick, rear leg

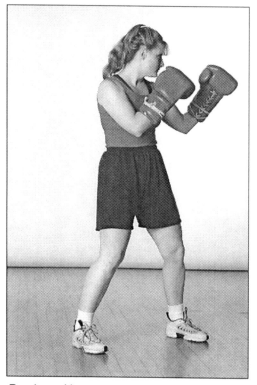

Ready position

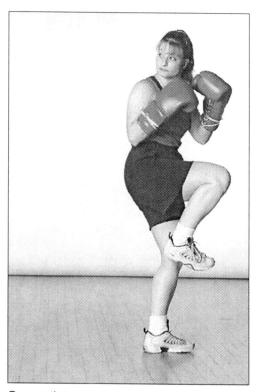

Preparation

Variation

Another variation for performing a rear kick with the front leg is to first take a small step or position the right foot (support leg) so that the foot is pointing at twelve noon as the target is sighted over the left shoulder. This is done prior to the preparatory phase of the rear kick. This variation is ideal when performing these kicks on a thick carpeted surface where pivoting may be difficult or for participants who have problems coordinating the pivoting movements on the balls of their feet.

Figure 4.32
Rear kick, rear leg; execution

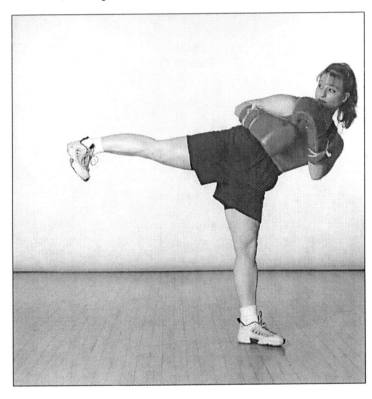

Knee Strikes

Knee strikes should be performed sparingly in an equipment-based class and contact should not be made directly on the patella. Knee strikes are best performed on a body shield because it can be manipulated at an angle so that contact is made with the flat portion of the upper thigh (proximal to the patella) when the knee joint is flexed. In this case, the participant pulls the top of the body shield toward his or her knee.

When using **Thai pads,** the participant closes the distance to the target in the preparation phase. The hands are placed on the holder's shoulders for balance only (Figure 4.33). To execute the

Figure 4.33
Knee strike

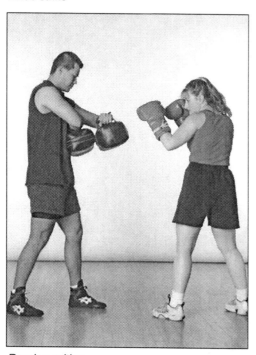

Ready position

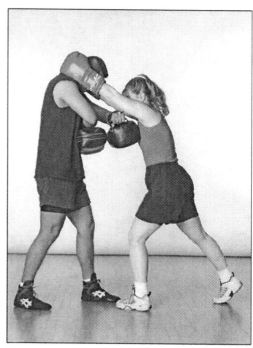

Preparation

knee strike, the rear leg (right knee and hip) is brought into flexion and the trunk is extended to maximize the impact of the strike. The foot of the support leg must have some external rotation as contact is made with the upper thigh (Figure 4.34). When using a body shield for a knee strike, the top portion is pulled down to knee-level as the knee strike is executed. Heavy bags are not the equipment of choice, but can be used if there is an ample amount of padding. When knee strikes are performed on a heavy bag, contact is made with the medial side of the knee.

Figure 4.34
Knee strike; execution

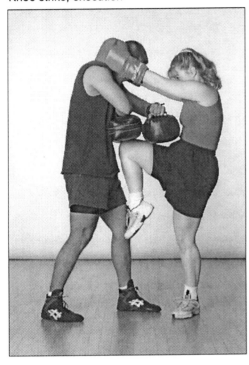

Proper Progression

The progression of punching or kicking at any level of intensity should be planned and graduated. If possible, develop separate classes and workouts for beginner, intermediate, and advanced participants. Beginning participants in equipment-based classes should devote their first workout to learning basic skills without any emphasis on power, speed, or use of equipment. Only during subsequent workouts should they be allowed to hit the heavy bag and use other equipment.

Limit combinations to no more than five total strikes, punches, or kicks. Keep in mind that the novice participant will be trying to learn and master new motor skills. Participants should find the workout challenging and not be struggling to keep up with the instructor. Select combinations that flow smoothly from one movement to the next and are as realistic as possible.

Injury Prevention

It would be ideal if all kickboxing participants had a high level of conditioning, as well as the appropriate muscular strength and endurance in the muscle groups used in a kickboxing workout. Since this is not realistic, you must plan each segment of the workout carefully. Because of the inherent risks, participants must ease into all movements. One of your priorities is to teach proper body

mechanics and limit or prevent participation in contact drills if you feel more time should be spent on the basics. Only participants with the appropriate conditioning and who have demonstrated proper mechanics should be punching or kicking with any speed or power. If appropriate, strikes with power as well as the number of power combinations should be dictated by the participants' level of training. Punching or kicking with the same arm or same leg should not be performed continuously for more than 30 seconds or 32 counts, and limit kicks to no more than 10 in a row for each leg. Also, remind participants to use the entire body when punching or kicking. When in doubt, keep the programming simple by incorporating basic combinations.

Floor Surfaces

A wooden floor is the ideal surface for kickboxing workouts because it offers the least amount of resistance to the rotational forces necessary to execute punches and kicks. If kickboxing must be taught on a carpeted surface, the carpet should be as thin as possible, and skills requiring pivoting movements such as left hooks and roundhouse kicks should be kept to a minimum.

High-risk and Contraindicated Movements

The skills performed in kickboxing are safe for most participants. However, certain skills may be considered high-risk depending on the skill, experience, and level of conditioning of the participant. Novice participants should avoid performing high kicks, punching with power, or performing a high number of repetitions with power or speed unless you are certain they can do so safely.

Sample Workouts

Equipment-based workouts

Sample Workout #1

Warm-up: Slow-speed shadowboxing

1st Round

(3-minute warm-up, 1-minute active rest)

• Hands: Jabs, straight rights, uppercuts, left hooks, elbow strikes

• Active rest: Squats, jump-rope drills without a rope

2nd Round

(3-minute warm-up, 1-minute active rest)

• Feet: Front kick, side kicks, rear kicks, roundhouse kicks, knee strikes

• Active rest: Squats, push-ups, crunches

3rd Round

(3-minute warm-up, 1-minute active rest)

• Hands and feet: Combinations of punches, kicks, elbow strikes, and knee strikes

• Active rest: Curl-ups and variations, single-leg raises

General Stretching: Major muscle groups

Conditioning: Bag work (2- to 3-minute rounds, 1-minute active rest periods)

Round 1: Jab to chin, right to chin (both sides)

Round 2: Jab to chin, right to chin, left hook to chin (both sides)

Round 3: Jab to chin, right to chin, left hook to chin, uppercut (both sides)

Conditioning: Thai pad/body shield (2-minute rounds, 1-minute active rest periods)

Round 1: Slow speed kicks, 30 seconds each leg

Round 2: Medium speed kicks, 30 seconds each leg

Round 3: Speed kicks with light power, 30 seconds each leg

Switch holders and repeat

Strengthening: Free weights and/or body weight

Cool-down

Stretching: Full-body stretching

Sample Workout # 2

Warm-up: Shadowboxing (5 minutes)

Stretching: 5 minutes

Conditioning: Shadow-kickboxing combinations (without equipment)

• Three to five movement combinations using both punches and kicks

• For each combination, perform two to three sets of eight to 10 repetitions

• Alternate right and left sides

• Active rest: Jumping jacks to increase heart rate or slow punches for recovery

Conditioning: Punching bag (15 to 20 minutes)

- Execute combinations from shadow-kickboxing drills or other combinations
- Work on form and rhythm
- 3 minutes each, 1-minute rest period

Strengthening: 10 minutes

Use of free weights and body weight

Cool-down: 5 minutes

Stretching: Full-body stretching

Non-equipment-based workouts

Sample Workout #3

Note:
- The individual exercises and moves can be repeated or cut down to vary the length of the workout.
- Moves and combinations are built around 32-count phrasing.
- Typically, one kick is performed every 4 counts, one punch is performed every 2 counts, and "tempo" punches are performed every 1 count (unless noted otherwise).

Warm-up:

March in place, four deep breaths, reaching overhead

Bob and weave with various arm patterns (each can be done for 32 counts):

1. on-guard position
2. on-guard position, alternate shoulder shrugs
3. reach/light jab in front, alternate arms (teach/review technique)
4. reach/light straight right, alternate arms (add foot pivot, teach/review technique)

- Step slide right and left, with arms in on-guard position

- Travel two steps right, then two steps left; add two right jabs while traveling right, two left jabs while traveling left
- *Warm-up combo:* Bob and weave right then left; add two shuffles/slide steps right; repeat bob and weave to the left then right; add two shuffles/slide steps left

Left leg lead: Teach/review left hook. Example:

1. on-guard position, lead leg pivots (16 counts)
2. add left elbow raise, parallel to floor (16 counts)
3. add full hook motion (32 counts)

Left leg lead: Teach/review right uppercut (32 counts each)

1. start with hip twist to front, right shoulder drop
2. add uppercut motion

Repeat both, right leg lead

Review front kicks: Example:

1. Right leg back, three lunges in place, right knee raise (repeat combination four times)
2. Repeat, changing right knee raise to right front kick (repeat combination four times)
3. Repeat steps 1 and 2 on the left leg

- Torso twists (on-guard position, twist side to side)
- Stretches for legs/arms/back

Cardio Segment:

Filler movements: Moves that can be put in between other moves and combos for various objectives, such as recovery time for other muscles, or to elevate the heart rate; usually done for 32-count intervals

1. Jumping rope (different variations)

2. Pummel run (tempo uppercut arms and wide leg stance)

3. Speed bag (one arm or both mimicking speed bag work while hopping, running, marching, standing)

4. Alternate punches at tempo, or short bursts of speedpunches

Set 1:

- Boxer's shuffle right and left, arms in on-guard position

- Left-leg lead shuffle front and back, add left jab (16 times)

- Shuffle right and left, add right jab to side (16 times)

- Repeat, alternating the two, reducing repetitions (eight times each, then four, then two; then alternate)

- Jump rope*

- Pummel run*

can be incorporated into combo, down to 4 counts each

Repeat jab combo, using right leg lead, right jabs

Set 2:

- Bob and weave

- Straight rights, varying tempos. Example:

1. Slow: Eight times, 4 counts each

2. 16 times, 2 counts each

- Repeat, using straight lefts

- Alternate straight rights and lefts (32–64 counts)

- Double up the straight rights and straight lefts, alternating between singles and doubles

- Alternate knee strikes (32 counts)

- Alternate front kicks (32 counts)

- Combo: Combine one knee and one kick (same leg or alternate right knee, left kick, etc.)

Set 3:

- Jump rope (32 counts)

- Alternate hooks (start with eight each, then alternate the two; reduce to two each)

- Alternate uppercuts (start with eight each, then alternate the two; reduce to two each)

- Elbow strikes variations (start with eight each, then alternate the two; reduce to two each)

Combo:

Alternate right and left hooks and uppercuts (4 counts)

Two right elbow strikes (4 counts)

Repeat, begin with left hook

Continue for total of 64 counts

Set 4:

- Right knee strikes (slow, then fast; 4 counts each) (32 counts)

- Right side kicks (slow, 8 counts, then singles at 4 counts each) (32 counts)

- Add a squat in between kicks

- Speed bag

- Repeat side knees and kicks on left leg

- Speed bag

- Alternate side kicks, right then left (4 counts each kick)

Set 5:

- Shuffle combos: Shuffle across the room with lead jabs three times, ending in straight rights (4 counts), and shuffle back to starting position
- Add on kicks/punches at the end, or change direction to forward/back
- Repeat/extend to raise heart rates

Set 6:

- One/two combo with knee and kick
- Left leg lead, left jab four times; straight right four times; reduce to alternate jab, straight right ("one/two") (4 counts)
- Speed it up to tempo, add hold in between; jab-cross (2 counts), hold (2 counts)
- Add one left jab (2 counts), then jab–straight right (left-right, 1 count each)
- Put together, add one right knee (2 counts), right kick (2 counts)
- Total of 8 counts
- Switch sides and repeat

Set 7:

- Body twist left; add three straight right knee strikes, one left jab; reduce to one knee, one straight right (repeat for 32 counts)

- Pummel run (repeat for 32 counts)
- Tempo: Alternate hooks or uppercuts set (32 counts)
- Repeat above combo to other side (begin with twist right)

  Or

- three straight rights, one right knee; kick from knee position
- Switch sides and repeat
- Tempo: Alternate hooks or uppercuts set (32 counts)

Set 8:

- Speed round of all punches:
  1. Left leg lead
  2. Left jab, straight right, left hook, right uppercut
  3. Start 2 counts each punch, go to tempo
  4. Repeat for 32 counts
- Switch sides and repeat

Cool-down/Floor:

- Slow movement: marching, lunging, etc.
- Stretching for larger leg muscles
- Push-ups, light weight work, etc.
- Abdominal work
- Stretch abs, arms, and legs

Bobbing and Weaving – Evading a series of punches through a combination of lateral movements and half squats.

Catching – A defensive movement of the hand(s) used against a left jab.

Ducking – A defensive movement that combines squatting and trunk flexion to duck a punch.

Equipment-based Workouts – Workouts that utilize equipment such as boxing gloves, heavy bags, kicking shields, Thai pads, etc.

Front Kick – A linear kick that is performed toward a target directly in front.

Jab – Punch with the non-dominant hand (usually the left for right-handers) that sets up all punches.

Knee Strikes – An offensive movement in which the rear leg is brought into flexion and the trunk is extended to maximum impact.

Left Hook – A short-range punch thrown in a circular motion that makes contact with the lateral side of the head or body.

Muay Thai – An ancient martial art; a precursor to modern kickboxing.

Non-equipment-based Workouts – Workouts that do not utilize any type of equipment.

On-guard Position – The proper hand positioning for both punching offense and defense.

Orthodox Stance – Basic stance for a right-handed individual; the left foot is in front and the right foot in back.

Parrying – Redirecting an oncoming punch by deflecting it.

Proprioception – Awareness of the body's position in space; helps the body regulate posture.

Rear Kick – A linear kick aimed at a target or opponent from the rear.

Roundhouse Kick – A circular kick that targets the lateral side of the head or body.

Side Kick – A linear kick that is performed toward a target or opponent from the side.

Slipping – Moving the trunk of the body to avoid a punch.

Southpaw Stance – Basic stance for a left-handed individual; the right foot is in front and the left foot in back.

Straight Right (Straight Left) – Power punch that uses the dominant hand and is thrown in a straight line.

Thai Pads – Kick pads; cover the forearm to absorb the shock of a kick or knee strike.

Uppercut – A punch thrown inside that usually targets the chin.

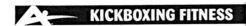
American College of Sports Medicine (2000). *ACSM's Guidelines for Exercise Testing and Prescription*, 6th Edition. Lippincott Williams & Wilkins.

American College of Sports Medicine. (1998). ACSM position stand on the recommended quantity and quality of exercise for developing and maintaining cardiorespiratory and muscular fitness, and flexibility in adults. *Medicine & Science in Sports & Exercise*, 30, 6, 975–991.

American College of Sports Medicine. (1997). *ACSM's Health/Fitness Facility Standards and Guidelines,* 2nd ed. Champaign, Ill.: Human Kinetics.

American Council on Exercise (1999). Cardio kickboxing packs a punch. *ACE FitnessMatters*. 5, 4, 4–5.

Bellinger, B. et al. (1997). Energy expenditure of a non-contact boxing training session compared with submaximal treadmill running. *Medicine & Science in Sports & Exercise*. 29, 12, 1653–1656.

Brown, J. *Ringside Boxing Manual.* Ringside, Inc.

National Sporting Goods Association (2003). Industry research and statistics; 2003 sports participation. www.nsga.org

Pitreli, J. & O'Shea, P. (1986). Sports Performance Series: Rope jumping: The biomechanics, techniques of and application to athletic conditioning. *National Strength and Conditioning Association*. 4, 5–13.

Quirk, J.E. & Sinning, W.E. (1982). Anaerobic and aerobic responses of males and females to rope skipping. *Medicine & Science in Sports & Exercise*. 14, 1, 26–29.

Solis, K. et al. (1988). Aerobic requirements for and heart rate responses to variations in rope jumping techniques. *Physician and Sports Medicine*. 16, 3, 121–128.

USA Boxing (2000). *Official Rules.*

Williams, A. (2000). Injury prevention in kickboxing classes. *IDEA Health and Fitness Source*. 18, 6, 63.

REFERENCES and Suggested Reading

ABOUT THE AUTHORS

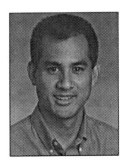

Tony Ordas, M.A., is a 4th degree black belt in Kenpo Karate and an active martial arts practitioner and instructor. He has a master's degree in Applied Exercise Physiology from San Diego State University and is an ACE-certified Personal Trainer, ACSM Exercise Specialist, and NSCA Certified Strength and Conditioning Specialist. Ordas, who was previously a clinical exercise physiologist at Scripps Clinic and certification director at ACE, has extensive experience developing exercise programs for cardiac rehabilitation, sport medicine, back rehabilitation, and weight management.

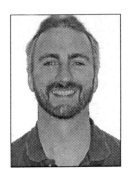

Tim Rochford, owner of Yorkville, Ill.–based Empower Training Systems, Inc., is a 5th degree black belt in Kajukenbo Karate and has been a sport karate and amateur kickboxing competitor since 1979. He holds personal trainer certifications from ACE, NASM, The Cooper Institute, AFAA, and NSCA, and is an ACE spokesperson for kickboxing fitness. Rochford, an adjunct instructor for The Cooper Institute and ACE continuing education specialist since 1995, was selected to the inaugural Board of Advisors for the American Council on Martial Arts in 1998.